TERESA SHIELDS PARKER

SWEET GRACE

STUDY GUIDE

**PRACTICAL STEPS
TO LOSE WEIGHT AND
OVERCOME SUGAR ADDICTION**

SWEET GRACE STUDY GUIDE

Printed in the USA

ISBN: 978-0-9910012-2-4

Library of Congress Control Number: 978-0-9910012-2-4

Published by Write the Vision | Columbia, Missouri

To Contact the Author:

www.teresashieldsparker.com

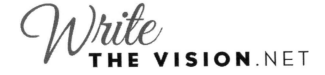

CONTENTS

6   Introduction

8   Who Am I?

10   Chapter 1—Sweet Grace

13   Chapter 2—Too Big For My Heart

17   Chapter 3—Comfort Food

21   Chapter 4—Snake In The Grass

25   Chapter 5—No Boundaries

28   Chapter 6—Eating Can Be Painful

31   Chapter 7—Time To Grow Up

35   Chapter 8—Trash Day Is So Romantic

38   Chapter 9—Hungry For It All

42   Chapter 10—In Search of Freedom

45   Chapter 11—Instant Pleasure

48   Chapter 12—Life Or Death

50   Chapter 13—Denial And Morbid Obesity

53   Chapter 14—Flip The Switch

57   Chapter 15—Breaking Sweet Chains

60   Chapter 16—Easy Button

63   Chapter 17—Power for the Powerless

67   Chapter 18—Grace, It's Not Just A Girl's Name

70   Chapter 19—Forgive

73   Chapter 20—Abundance

76   Action Steps

89   Covenant

93   Photo Pages

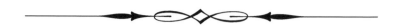

INTRODUCTION

When I wrote my memoir, *Sweet Grace: How I Lost 250 Pounds and Stopped Trying To Earn God's Favor*, I included questions at the end of each chapter. I wrote the book to share my story and to provide hope, especially to the morbidly obese individuals, as well as anyone caught in addiction of any sort.

Many who helped me by reading the book before publication shared their desire to read the story through first and then think about the implications. This bothered me a bit because what good is it if I share my story, but no one learns the lessons of how an over-emphasis on food, or anything else for that matter, can ruin a person's life?

I believe in the necessity of studying what you read. So I put together this *Sweet Grace Study Guide* to include basic steps for becoming healthy, thought-provoking questions, study questions related to each chapter, personal applications and space to journal, draw, create and ponder all the issues brought up in the book.

If you are doing the study with a group, read each chapter and complete the study guide for the chapter. Then share your answers with the group. This is a bit of a different kind of study guide. Each session includes some creative endeavors, as well as activities designed to help you learn to be whole, healthy and happy.

After you finish working through the questions and activities related to the memoir, there are 12 Action Steps to help you get started on your journey towards health. Each action step includes more questions all designed to help you move forward on your journey. In my opinion, this is one of the most critical pieces of the study guide. Take your time doing this. If you are studying with a group, do an action step each session. Make sure everyone is on board with the completion of the step and they know where they are headed.

Let me say here, do not think you or everyone in your group has to change their lifestyle overnight. For some, it will happen that way. For others, small steps done well and completely are vitally important. Celebrate where everyone is and how quickly they want to move. Encourage and uplift each other. Never place shame or guilt on others or yourself. This is critical in the weight loss and healthy eating journey.

I remember when I was extremely overweight, one slip-up would make me feel like giving up and so I would. I would think I'm doomed. I can't do this. Might as well eat what I really want to eat. And I'd be off on a binge that might take years to come out of, if even then. Accept yourself and every person in your group for where they are and who they are. If they never lose a pound, they are still beautiful, loveable and wonderful just like they are. God sees us this way and we surely need to see ourselves and others this way.

This study could be foundational for some people. It could plant a seed that may not grow until a few years down the road. Every effort we make to learn and become healthy will be beneficial no matter if we do a total turnaround or not. I encourage you to give yourself some grace in the process. Grace is the nature of God.

Finally, I've included an outline to help you develop a personal covenant, a kind of stake in the ground to mark your decisions. As promised, at the end are some photos. I included them because you asked for them!

If you are doing this in a group, each member should have a copy of the memoir, *Sweet Grace* and this study guide. Do not try to do this study without reading or listening to the memoir. It is available on Amazon in paperback, kindle and audible.

Leaders should look at each lesson and decide which activities your group will do together at your meeting. Let your members know the plan for the next meeting. For group activities, let members know if they need to bring anything. Many activities have suggestions for group activities. All are easily adapted.

My heart goes with you as you engage in this study. Talking about health and weight issues can be heavy (excuse the pun). It is true, though, because it cuts deep to the heart and self-image of any man or woman. I did write the study guide with women in mind, but I am well aware that many men suffer with these same issues. You may wish to open your study to men, as well.

Feel free to connect with me at teresa@writethevision.net if you have any questions about the study. Let me know how it goes.

Now, buckle your seat belts. It's going to be a wild ride.

—Teresa Shields Parker

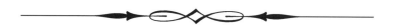

WHO AM I?

Since you took time to read my book, I thought I'd take a moment and introduce myself. I'm Teresa Shields Parker and I have lost 263 pounds and hope to lose at least 18 more to get me in the "normal" weight range, whatever that is. Since you read my memoir, obviously you know way more about me than I know about you.

I'll just share a bit that you may not know. I love Britt Nicole's song, *All This Time*, because from the moment I met the Lord as a child of seven, through every good and every bad choice of my life, He has been walking with me, leading me gently by His grace. My eyes get misty just thinking about the grace He poured out on me even in spite of my failures.

Although there are many nouns that describe what I do, they don't really describe who I am. I decided back in 1994 that I wanted to be a whole, healthy, happy woman of God. And although I am not quite there yet, I am much closer than I was when I said that almost 20 years ago.

It is from that life focus that I write, edit and publish stories that connect people to their destiny in the Creator. What I have that helps me write is a bachelor's degree in journalism and a master's degree in Biblical studies.

Personally, my husband, Roy, and I have been married for 36 years and are more in love now than ever before. We have two grown children, Jenny and Andrew. Currently, Jenny lives in Japan where she teaches English. Andrew is a wandering computer technician currently residing with us. Two grand-cats, Harley and Fluff, rule the roost while Jenny and Andrew roam the world.

We have a business taking care of developmentally challenged young women. We're busy, in other words, probably like most of you. We are active members of a growing contemporary charismatic congregation. I am active in the communications, women's and life group ministries there. Of course, I'm partial to the life group I lead in my home. My LOL girls keep me sane in an insane world.

The most important thing about me, though, is that I can finally say God is my all. He is first without a second in my life. I learn more about Him every day as I grow closer and closer to Him.

I've learned that He left His Holy Spirit here for three purposes—to comfort, teach and nurture us. I don't know about you, but I looked for comfort in food, mainly sugar and bread, for years before I really understood that the best comfort available dwelt inside of me. I love that He has our best interests at heart and wants us to be whole, healthy and happy even more than we do.

My desire is that this study will touch your heart and life. I want you to think, ponder, create, laugh, cry and take action. Most of all, I want the precious Holy Spirit to invade your life with grace and truth in a way you've never experienced before.

RESPOND

If you were to meet me for the first time, what would you tell me about yourself? Who is your family? Where do you work? What are your passions? What is unique about you? Who are you? Journal your response to this and other questions throughout the study.

What would you like to get out of this study?

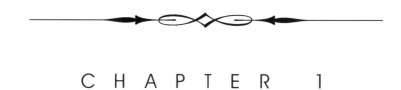

CHAPTER 1

SWEET GRACE

READ CHAPTER 1, SWEET GRACE.

THINK ABOUT IT

Read the "Who am I" section. What song speaks to you especially regarding your spiritual journey?

What verse, phrase or word in the song really shouts at you and why?

Using the first chapter of *Sweet Grace* as a guide of sorts, write about your journey with God. When did you realize you were in need of God's grace? How did you come to know Him?

How has God made a difference in your life today?

READ AND WRITE

"For it is by grace you have been saved, through faith—and this is not from yourselves, it is the gift of God—not by works, so that no one can boast." Ephesians 2:8-9, NIV

What is the meaning of "grace" in this scripture?

What is the meaning of "works" in that scripture?

What does the phrase "not by works, so that no one can boast" mean to you personally? How do you see this playing out in your life?

CREATE

Draw a picture depicting what God means to you.

ACT

Talk to an elderly relative or another elderly individual who is a Christian. Ask them what has been the best thing about walking with God all this time. If you are working with a group, ask the oldest person in the group to answer this question and so on, to the youngest.

FOLLOW-THROUGH

Journal about who you interviewed and what you learned here.

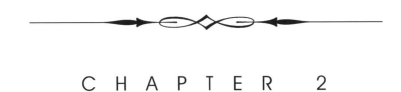

C H A P T E R   2

TOO BIG FOR MY HEART

READ CHAPTER 2, TOO BIG FOR MY HEART.

THINK ABOUT IT

Sometimes we pervert foods that taste good into foods in which we overindulge. Why do we do this?

Do you think it is something we consciously choose to do? If so, why?

How does overindulgence affect you while you are indulging? After you indulge?

READ AND WRITE

"He replied, 'Because you have so little faith. Truly I tell you, if you have faith as small as a mustard seed, you can say to this mountain, 'Move from here to there,' and it will move. Nothing will be impossible for you.'" Matthew 17:20, NIV

What is faith to you?

For what do you have faith? List these. Be specific.

List the things for which you don't have faith. Be specific.

Why do you think you don't have faith for those things?

What challenges do you have regarding faith?

"Today I have given you the choice between life and death, between blessings and curses. I call on heaven and earth to witness the choice you make. Oh, that you would choose life, that you and your descendants might live! Choose to love the Lord your God and to obey Him and commit yourself to Him, for He is your life. Then you will live long in the land the Lord swore to give your ancestors Abraham, Isaac, and Jacob." Deuteronomy 30:19-20, NLT

In what ways do you choose life? Be specific.

In what ways do you choose death? Be specific.

What does it mean to really live?

What would it look like? Be specific about what it would involve or contain.

What has been the biggest turning point in your life?

CREATE

Write your obituary as if you died today.

Write your obituary as if you lived to be 100. Incorporate the things you have changed to make your life better.

ACT

Interview someone of the same gender that you really admire. Ask them, " If you could change one thing about your life, what would it be?" If you are working as a group, divide into pairs and interview each other. Take notes on the interview. Ask questions.

FOLLOW-THROUGH

Journal about the interview and what you learned. You might want to write a short feature story about your interview.

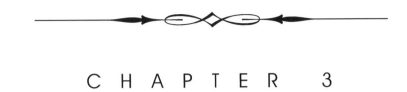

CHAPTER 3

COMFORT FOOD

READ CHAPTER 3, COMFORT FOOD.

THINK ABOUT IT

I love the song, "It Is Well." When all is not well with my soul, listening to lyrics and a gentle melody that say just the opposite really helps. You may go in an entirely different direction when you are stressed. What song brings you comfort and why?

Where do you find comfort? Where do you turn when you are hurting, sick, scared or sad? What comforts work for you and don't work for you?

Is there anything you always go to for comfort? Is there anything you go to for comfort that has gotten out of control? Why do you think that is?

In a recent survey taken by beliefnet.com, sweets were the number one type of comfort food, followed by warm, salty, cheesy and/or fresh food. Does it surprise you that sweets would rank highest as a comfort food? Why do you think that is?

READ AND WRITE

"Now we see things imperfectly, like puzzling reflections in a mirror, but then we will see everything with perfect clarity. All that I know now is partial and incomplete, but then I will know everything completely, just as God now knows me completely." 1 *Corinthians 13:12, NLT*

What role did food play in your home growing up? How did your parents view food, supper, and snacks?

When did you receive food as a reward? How does that impact you today?

How was food used as a comfort? What types of food? Who prepared these?

Do you use food as a comfort today? How? What foods?

CREATE

This activity makes a great group activity. However, you can also do it on your own. It does take some time to do so if you are doing it as a group. Set aside at least an hour from start to finish.

Make a Vision Board about what you would like in your life in this season. Vision boards can actually call up what's on the inside of you in an almost prophetic way. I made my first Vision Board about a year before I finished writing this book. At the time the book was in the back of my mind. As I sit here looking at my board I think it's so interesting that the only pictures on the board are books. Some of the prime phrases are Believe. Living Your best Life. The Writer's House. Life-Changing Journey. Energy. The Storyteller. Happiness. Be Healthy. Live Healthy. Grace. Truth. Now if that doesn't sum up my book, I'm not sure what does.

A small poster board works well for this exercise. Gather old magazines, newspapers, scraps of material, colored paper, as well as markers, glue, scissors and tape. It really is best to set a time limit for this project and not to over think it.

Go through the magazines and newspapers and tear or cut out pictures and phrases that speak to you. Look through the other items you have gathered and choose things you'd like to add to your collage. Your theme will develop as you find the items that speak to something deep inside you. Arrange your items on the board. Glue or tape them down. Use the markers to add words if you wish.

What is the theme of your board? What did you learn from creating it?

Display your board in a place where you can see it often. Next year, look back and learn from the Vision you had for the year.

ACT

Think of one comfort food you love. How could you re-create this food so it was healthy? Go online and search for similar healthy recipes or attempt to create your own. What can you cook up? Record your healthy recipe here.

FUN

Prepare your recipe and invite some people over to enjoy it. If you are working with a group, prepare the recipe for a group session.

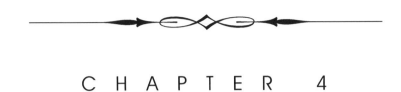

CHAPTER 4

SNAKE IN THE GRASS

READ CHAPTER 4, SNAKE IN THE GRASS.

THINK ABOUT IT

One of my favorite songs is "You'll Get Through This" by Martina McBride. Search for it on YouTube, find it and play it. The chorus says simply, "You'll get through this. No matter what it takes. I believe in you for heaven's sake. You'll get through this." I do wish Martina had written that song and I had heard it when I was 11. There was the feeling I would not get through the shame I felt by what Fred did.

Is there a similar song that speaks to you about a difficult time in your life when you didn't think you would make it? What is the song and why does it speak to you?

What do you do when you want to do as McBride sings, "Pull the shades down on the sun. Don't want to see the morning break to another day I don't have the strength to face. Close the door and keep it shut. Lord, this ache is just too much for me to take. How do I begin to pray?" In other words, what gets you through to the next day and why? Be honest.

READ AND WRITE

"For all have sinned and fall short of the glory of God and are justified freely by His grace through the redemption that came by Christ Jesus." Romans 3:23-24, NIV

Fred was an every Sunday church member. What part do you think God's grace, as mentioned in Romans 3:23-24, plays in the case of the Freds out there sitting in the church pews?

Was there a time you were abused sexually, physically or verbally? Write about it and how it made you feel.

What did you do about it at the time?

Imagine you are back in that situation at the age you were then. If you could rewrite how you responded during the situation or afterwards, would there have been anything you would change?

How did the incident affect your life after that time?

What bearing did the abuse have on your relationship with food?

CREATE

Paint a picture depicting how you have felt powerless and used in a situation. In the same picture, add a part that shows you having power over the powerless situation. It can be arranged or depicted any way you wish. It can be abstract, realistic, futuristic or stick figures. Use acrylic paints on canvas board, watercolor on watercolor paper, color markers on heavy paper or colored pencil on paper. If you wish, find a scripture that gives you hope and note it somewhere in your painting or drawing. Make sure it is something you can save with your Study Guide items or display in a place you can see, in order to know there is hope even in powerless situations. If you are meeting with a group, decide if you are doing this together or on your own and then share the picture with the group.

What did you learn from creating your painting or drawing?

ACT

Find a local children's and women's shelter or crisis center and volunteer to help in some way. It may be as simple as collecting food or clothing or as involved as completing an application to become a volunteer. If you are meeting with a group, schedule a time to do this together.

FOLLOW-THROUGH

Journal about what you did, what happened and what you learned.

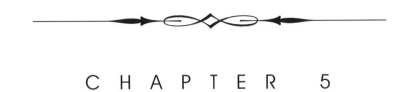

CHAPTER 5

NO BOUNDARIES

READ CHAPTER 5, NO BOUNDARIES

THINK ABOUT IT

Perhaps you have a vision, dream, goal or destiny to which you feel called. Maybe God has actually tapped you on the shoulder and asked you to step up to the plate in some area. However, there is something standing in the way of your dream. You can't put your finger on it, but you know you are impeding the progress. I know this all too well. I was clinging to something that had no value. I wanted what God wanted for me, but I also wanted what was in the way.

The song that speaks of this so well is "Dreams I Dream For You" by Avalon. If you have the capability, search for it on You Tube and play it. Otherwise, search for the lyrics. They are an important part of this chapter.

Here is the chorus, "The dreams I dream for you are deeper that the ones you're clinging to. More precious than the finest things you knew and truer than the treasures you pursue. Let the old dreams die like stars that fade from view. Then take the cup I offer and drink deeply of the dreams I dream for you."

What is the most important thing in your life right now? If there was one thing you would not give up what would it be? If God asked you to give that up for the dream He has for you, would you do it? Why or why not?

What is God's dream or vision for your life as you understand it today?

How do we sometimes get sidetracked from pursuing God's dream for our lives?

How has food replaced a dream or vision for your life?

READ AND WRITE

"Like a city whose walls are broken through is a person who lacks self-control."
Proverbs 25:28, NIV

What are your walls or boundaries? List these. Be specific. What things are you willing to do or not do?

Do your walls need to be repaired? If so, where do they need to be repaired? How can you repair them?

"Now you know full well the doings of our lower natures. Fornication, impurity, indecency, idol-worship, sorcery; enmity, strife, jealousy, outbursts of passion, intrigues, dissensions, factions, envyings; hard drinking, riotous feasting, and the like. And as to these I forewarn you, as I have already forewarned you, that those who are guilty of such things will have no share in the Kingdom of God." Galatians 5:19-21, Weymouth New Testament.

This passage of scripture discusses some of the deeds of the flesh. What are the deeds of the flesh do you struggle with, and what causes you to gravitate towards these things.

ACT

Research one aspect of a dream that is in your heart. Read a book on the subject, search the topic on the internet, investigate local college classes, apply to a college, update your resume and/or apply for a job you've always wanted. If you are working in a group, share this with them. If not, note it here.

CREATE

Draw a picture of a boundary in your life and the breach or the difficulty that keeps that boundary from being firm.

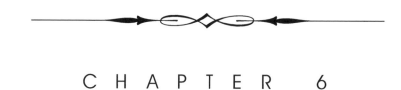

CHAPTER 6

EATING CAN BE PAINFUL

READ CHAPTER 6, EATING CAN BE PAINFUL.

THINK ABOUT IT

In life, many things call to us that aren't necessarily helpful. It is a little like the verse, "What does it profit a man (or woman) who gains the whole world but loses his (or her) soul?" Of course Toby Mac, Kirk Franklin and Mandisa say it better in the song, "Lose My Soul."

There's a lot to think about in this song. The basic message is the same as the scripture. "I don't want to gain the whole world and lose my soul." At the end of the first verse, it says, "Everything that I see draws me, though it's only in You that I can truly see that it's a feast for the eyes—a low blow to purpose. And I'm a little kid at a three ring circus."

What are some things that seem good at the time, but actually have the possibility of drawing you away from God or as the song puts it are "a low blow to purpose"? List these. Be specific.

What causes you anxiety or stress and what do you do when you have anxiety or stress? How do you relieve it?

READ AND WRITE

"Trust God from the bottom of your heart; don't try to figure out everything on your own. Listen for God's voice in everything you do, everywhere you go; He's the one who will keep you on track. Don't assume that you know it all. Run to God! Run from evil! Your body will glow with health, your very bones will vibrate with life!" Proverbs 3:5-8 MSG

What is the difference between trusting God and figuring things out on your own?

How does God keep you on track? Or how do you keep on track with God?

How are physical and spiritual health related?

REFLECT

Make a stress chart. List stressors starting with the thing that causes you the most stress to the least. Then beside each stressor list what your go-to resource is to relieve that stress. In the third column list a more healthy way to relieve the stress. Be specific about each column. In the third column, list some specific action, hobby or activity.

Stressor	Go-To Reliever	Healthy Stress Reliever
1.		
2.		
3.		
4.		
5.		
6.		
7.		
8.		
9.		
10.		

ACT

Make a Healthy Stress Reliever box. On 3x5 cards list one stress reliever idea with any additional information you need to engage in that activity, such as where supplies are kept. When you are tempted to go to food, go to your Healthy Stress Reliever box instead. Add special scriptures that have been meaningful to you. If you are working with a group, make your 3x5 cards together, brainstorming and sharing ideas as you go. When you get home find and decorate a recipe box or some other box to hold your cards.

FUN

Choose one of the items you put in the "Healthy Stress Reliever" column and do this activity. If you are working with a group, nominate some of the ideas, vote and choose one to do as a group.

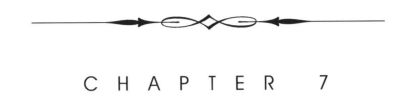

CHAPTER 7

TIME TO GROW UP

READ CHAPTER 7, TIME TO GROW UP

THINK ABOUT IT

When I was a kid I disliked the song, "Jesus Loves Me." I think it's because we sang it every single Sunday. I went to a church where the pianist and organist dueled each other with lively gospel music. I loved worshipping with the adults because their music was much more fun than "Jesus Loves Me" which seemed to be three times as long as any worship song we sang in the adult service. It wasn't until I was an adult that I really understand that "Jesus Loves Me" had a much deeper message than just a song for kindergartners. Any song that declares Jesus' love is very special.

What are some songs you sang as a child. List these. What did they mean to you then and what do the mean to you now?

Do you have a significant person in your life that doesn't understand your issues with food? How do you deal with this?

In what ways have discussion about food meant one thing to you and another to someone significant to you?

If you are married, in what ways did you assume all your worries were over when you got married? If you are single, in what ways do you assume all your worries will be over when you get married?

READ AND WRITE

"When I was a child, I talked like a child, I spoke and thought and reasoned as child. But when I grew up, I put away childish things." 1 Corinthians 13:11, NLT

What does this scripture mean to you? Is it possible all the time? When is it not possible?

How can you put away childish things, especially as it relates to food, if the tug is emotionally ingrained?

Do you have issues from your childhood that have reared their ugly heads in adulthood? How do you deal with these issues?

Write about a time in your adulthood that you responded to a difficulty in a childish way.

CREATE

In the space below using a pencil or colored markers, on one half of the page, draw a picture of yourself as a child, any age you choose doing anything you choose. Now, with the hand you don't normally write with, draw another picture of yourself on the other half of the paper. If you are right-handed, do it left-handed. Don't try to laboriously copy the picture. You can draw the same picture, but allow it to come as that hand wishes it to come. In other words, let it flow. Now with the same hand that drew the picture write a caption below each picture.

What is the difference between the two pictures you drew? Do you feel any differently drawing the pictures? Are the captions the same or different? Why did you put the captions you did?

Research shows that no matter which hand we favor in writing or drawing, if we use the other hand it gives greater access to right hemisphere functions like feeling, intuition, creativity, inner wisdom and spirituality. Some say this is true no matter which is our non-dominant hand. Others say it helps us get in touch with the inner child.

FUN

Try this same activity with some children in your life, just for fun. Do they care as much about the result of the non-dominant hand as you did?

FOLLOW-THROUGH

Journal about what you did, what happened and what you learned here.

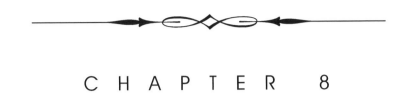

CHAPTER 8

TRASH DAY IS SO ROMANTIC

READ CHAPTER 8, TRASH DAY IS SO ROMANTIC

THINK ABOUT IT

One of my favorite love songs is "Evergreen" by Barbara Streisand. And yes, it *was* played at my wedding. "Two lights that shine as one, morning glory and the midnight sun. Time, we've learned to sail above. Time won't change the meaning of one love. Ageless and ever, evergreen." I love the song, but if I really analyze it I probably wouldn't agree with every part. When I was young, I believed in a romantic love where everything was perfect every day. However, after 36 years of marriage, I realize that everything is not perfect and because of that it's awesome to have someone special to share the good times and the bad times with. I do believe this part, though, love is ageless and new at the same time.

What is you favorite love song and why? What do you agree with and disagree with in the song?

Has your marriage or a significant relationship ever been in trouble because of your weight? How did you handle this?

What happens when someone suggests you should lose weight? Write about a time this has happened.

If you wanted to lose weight, how could a loved one support you in that effort?

How are anger, control and other emotional issues, related to food?

READ AND WRITE

"They willfully put God to the test by demanding the food they craved ... They ate the bread of angels; He sent them all the food they could eat." Psalm 78:18 & 25, NIV

Why did God grant the Israelites' prayer?

"If anyone, then, knows the good they ought to do and doesn't do it, it is sin for them." James 4:17, NIV

Is there anything you are currently doing that you know is not what God would consider "good" for you or for your relationship with Him? List these things.

Are you willing to lay these things down? If so write out a prayer of surrender to God. Spend some time sharing your heart with Him. Write your prayer out here.

ACT

Buy groceries for someone or prepare food of some kind and take it to someone just because. If you are working with a group, do this together.

FOLLOW-THROUGH

Journal about what you did, who you did it for, what happened and what you learned.

CREATE

Write a story from the point of view of a husband who would like to help his wife lose weight. What is he thinking? What does he do right? What does he do wrong? Show it in the story. If you are working with a group, share your story.

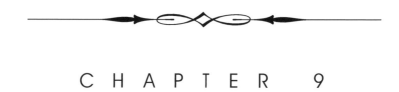

CHAPTER 9

HUNGRY FOR IT ALL

READ CHAPTER 9, HUNGRY FOR IT ALL

THINK ABOUT IT

Are you super woman or do you feel the need to be? Peggy Lee's priceless song, "I'm A Woman" talks about this. If you search for the words to the song, though, they don't include: "I can bring home the bacon and fry it up in a pan." That actually was a revamped 80s version for an Enjoli commercial. Peggy's version says: "I can scoop up a great big dipper full of lard from the drippins can, throw it in the skillet, go out and do my shopping, be back before it melts in the pan." You get my drift.

As women, we get the idea we should be super women and not only can, but have to do it all. Do you see this super woman syndrome as a trait of gender or of culture or both? What's good about it? What's bad about it?

How has the church encouraged this "super woman syndrome"?

How has the "super woman sydrome" affected you?

READ AND WRITE

"A wife of noble character who can find? She is worth far more than rubies. Her husband has full confidence in her and lacks nothing of value. She brings him good, not harm, all the days of her life. She selects wool and flax and works with eager hands. She is like the merchant ships, bringing her food from afar. She gets up while it is still night; she provides food for her family and portions for her female servants. She considers a field and buys it; out of her earnings she plants a vineyard. She sets about her work vigorously; her arms are strong for her tasks. She sees that her trading is profitable and her lamp does not go out at night. In her hand she holds the distaff and grasps the spindle with her fingers. She opens her arms to the poor and extends her hands to the needy. When it snows, she has no fear for her household; for all of them are clothed in scarlet. She makes coverings for her bed; she is clothed in fine linen and purple. Her husband is respected at the city gate, where he takes his seat among the elders of the land. She makes linen garments and sells them, and supplies the merchants with sashes. She is clothed with strength and dignity; she can laugh at the days to come. She speaks with wisdom, and faithful instruction is on her tongue. She watches over the affairs of her household and does not eat the bread of idleness. Her children arise and call her blessed; her husband also, and he praises her: Many women do noble things, but you surpass them all. Charm is deceptive, and beauty is fleeting; but a woman who fears the Lord is to be praised. Honor her for all that her hands have done, and let her works bring her praise at the city gate." Proverbs 31:10-31, NIV

What is this passage really trying to say to women? What does it say to you?

'There is no fear in love; but perfect love casts out fear, because fear involves torment. But he who fears has not been made perfect in love." 1 John 4:18, NKJV

"The fear of the Lord is the beginning of knowledge." Proverbs 1:7 NIV

"The fear of the Lord is the beginning of wisdom, and knowledge of the Holy One is understanding." Proverbs 9:10, NIV

What does fearing the Lord mean to you?

"The angel of the Lord encamps around those who fear Him, and He delivers them. Taste and see that the Lord is good ; blessed is the man who takes refuge in Him."
Psalm 34:7-8, NIV

What does it mean to taste and see that the Lord is good?

"Blessed are those who hunger and thirst for righteousness, for they will be filled."
Matthew 5:6, NIV

How can we be as hungry for God as we are for food?

"For you created my inmost being; You knit me together in my mother's womb. I praise You because I am fearfully and wonderfully made; Your works are wonderful, I know that full well. My frame was not hidden from You when I was made in the secret place, when I was woven together in the depths of the earth. Your eyes saw my unformed body; all the days ordained for me were written in Your book before one of them came to be." Psalm 139: 13-16, NIV

Many times we think we have to be more than who we were actually created to be. What does this passage lead you to believe about yourself?

"'Did someone bring Him food while we were gone?' the disciples asked each other."
John 4:33, NLT

Where should we get our nourishment? How does this play out in your life?

What are some healthy ways we can re-fuel ourselves when we feel like we are running on empty?

CREATE

Write your own version of Proverbs 31:10-31. Make it a modern day reflection of where you are at right now. It doesn't have to follow the scriptures exactly. Let it flow from where you are.

ACT

Volunteer to help a single mother in some way. Watch her children. Prepare a meal for her. Help her create a resume to find a better job. Help her find work clothes. Ask her what she needs that you could help her with. If you are working with a group, do this together.

FOLLOW-THROUGH

Journal about what you did, when you did it, who was there, what happened, what you learned here and why it was fun.

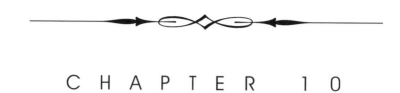

CHAPTER 10

IN SEARCH OF FREEDOM

READ CHAPTER 10, IN SEARH OF FREEDOM

THINK ABOUT IT

When I was in high school one of my favorite artists was Rod Stewart. "Reason to Believe" was released when I was a junior dreaming about the love of my life, whom I hadn't met yet. Even though it was a song about love and broken hearts and all of that, I loved the line, "Still I look to find a reason to believe." That song summed up a lot of my life. Though I was a Christian I still questioned everything and looked to find reasons to believe all the time. It's a core value of my life that I don't take things at face value, but I had not applied it to myself.

I realized just recently how much that song applies to me. What I decided back in 1994 was that I wanted to be a writer who makes a difference in the lives of others. In order to have what I wanted, I needed to be a whole, healthy, happy woman. I would did not really start to become that until I found a reason to believe in myself as much or more than anyone else.

What about you? What singers or groups did you follow in high school? What song or lyric still sticks in your mind? What connection might it have to what you want? If you don't know the answer to the last question, just jot down the name of an artist, song and a lyric. You can figure out the rest later.

What is a dream of yours that you've always had? Perhaps it's a dream that's been in the back of your mind since you were a child. State it here simply.

As an adult what do you want? Describe a dream you'd like to fulfill or some specific goal you'd like to reach. Don't worry about whether it is attainable or not. Just list the dream or dreams.

What kind of person would have what you want? What type of person would attain your dream? What would be their attributes? Would they be strong, brave, healthy, creative, joyful, engaging, peaceful? There are thousands of words you could choose from. List those that come to your mind. It's OK if it's just one word or several words.

What kinds of things might you have to discard from your life to be that kind of person?

What would have to happen for you to be free of those things that keep you from being the kind of person that can have what you want?

READ AND WRITE

"And you shall know the truth, and the truth will set you free." John 8:32, NKJV

What is the truth about yourself that God sees?

What is the truth about yourself that you need to see and understand?

How would embracing that set you free?

CREATE

Using markers, colored pencils or crayons draw a picture of freedom. It could just be words that describe that to you.

ACT

Find a song from your high school years that encourages you to be the person you want to be. It will probably be a song that was one you really liked during those years. Learn the words. Dress up like the artist who sang that song, cue up a version of the song and lip sync it for some friends or if you are meeting with a group, do it together as a group. Share why this song is meaningful to you. Most of all, have fun. Then list the feelings you had while doing this.

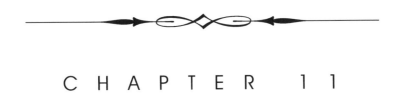

CHAPTER 11

INSTANT PLEASURE

READ CHAPTER 11, INSTANT PLEASURE

THINK ABOUT IT

Let's suppose scientists have created a pill that gives instant pleasure. The pleasure sensation lasts for only five minutes. There are no known side effects. If given the chance, would you volunteer for testing? Why or why not?

To my knowledge this kind of pill has not been developed, but if it was what would be some of the advantages?

What would be the disadvantages?

What are some of the things we use to bring instant pleasure?

In your opinion, are these good or bad? Necessary or unnecessary?

READ AND WRITE

"Let us then approach God's throne of grace with confidence, so that we may receive mercy and find grace to help us in our time of need." Hebrews 4:16, NIV

When have you gone to God in a time of need? How did He help you?

"Praise be to the God and Father of our Lord Jesus Christ, who has blessed us in the heavenly realms with every spiritual blessing in Christ." Ephesians 1:3, NIV

"Which of you, if your son asks for bread, will give him a stone? Or if he asks for a fish, will give him a snake? If you, then, though you are evil, know how to give good gifts to your children, how much more will your Father in heaven give good gifts to those who ask Him!" Matthew 7:9-11, NIV

"Why, my soul, are you downcast? Why so disturbed within me? Put your hope in God, for I will yet praise Him, my Savior and my God." Psalm 42:5, NIV

"For we do not have a high priest who is unable to empathize with our weaknesses, but we have One who has been tempted in every way, just as we are—yet He did not sin." Hebrews 4:15, NIV

What are some things God has promised to do for you? List these from the scriptures above. Add others if you wish.

"I do not understand what I do. For what I want to do I do not do, but what I hate I do. And if I do what I do not want to do, I agree that the law is good. As it is, it is no longer I myself who do it, but it is sin living in me. For I know that good itself does not dwell in me, that is, in my sinful nature. For I have the desire to do what is good, but I cannot carry it out. For I do not do the good I want to do, but the evil I do not want to do—this I keep on doing. Now if I do what I do not want to do, it is no longer I who do it, but it is sin living in me that does it. So I find this law at work: although I want to do good, evil is right there with me. For in my inner being I delight in God's law; but I see another law at work in me, waging war against the law of my mind and making me a prisoner of the law of sin at work within me. What a wretched man I am! Who will rescue me from this body that is subject to death?" Romans 7:15-24, NIV

What does this passage say to you in regard to compulsive overeating?

"What causes fights and quarrels among you? Don't they come from your desires that battle within you? You desire but do not have, so you kill. You covet but you cannot get what you want, so you quarrel and fight. You do not have because you do not ask God. When you ask, you do not receive, because you ask with wrong motives, that you may spend what you get on your pleasures. You adulterous people, don't you know that friendship with the world means enmity against God? Therefore, anyone who chooses to be a friend of the world becomes an enemy of God." James 4:1-4, NIV

Does this passage speak to you regarding compulsive overeating? If so, how?

ACT

Plan a party without unhealthy food. If you have food, what will it be? What will you do for activities? What will you do for fun? Have the party. Take a video of the activities. Share on social media. If you are working with a group, do this together.

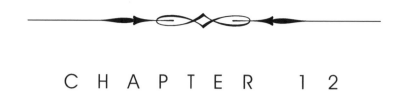

C H A P T E R   1 2

LIFE OR DEATH

READ CHAPTER 12, LIFE OR DEATH

THINK ABOUT IT

Have you tried breaking the chain of your food issue yourself? In what ways did this work? What ways did it not work?

Have you tried having another person help you with your food issue? Who and when? How did this work or not work?

Have you tried a treatment program of some kind? What worked? What didn't work?

READ AND WRITE

"And behold, an angel of the Lord suddenly appeared and a light shone in the cell; and he struck Peter's side and woke him up, saying, 'Get up quickly.' And his chains fell off his hands." Acts 12:7, NASB

In what ways is your food issue like being in prison or like being chained?

What do you think would be your God-sized intervention, one which would allow the chains to simply fall off like they did for Peter?

CREATE

Make a chain out of construction paper. Cut strips of paper. Write various things you are in bondage to on each slip of paper. It could be various types of food, drink, activities, television shows or other things. Using glue or tape, make a chain by securing one end of the strip to the other. Loop the next link through and secure it. Making this a large chain will give you a physical idea of the bondage you are in.

ACT

Using the chain you have, read each word and give it to God. Ask Him to break the chains in your life that the words on the chain represent. Then, break the chain and tear it up. Burn it in a fireplace or outdoor fire pit or put it in a garbage can. If you are working with a group, this will be a meaningful activity to do together.

FUN

As a group, celebrate your life and freedom together. Make sure it is a celebration that doesn't lead anyone in your group back into bondage or temptation. Brainstom some things you could do. Then plan a time to do them. Journal about what you did and how it was fun for you without temptation.

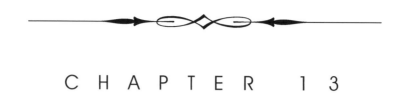

CHAPTER 13

DENIAL AND MORBID OBESITY

READ CHAPTER 13, DENIAL AND MORBID OBESITY

THINK ABOUT IT

Denial is a fascinating subject. It is actually a defense mechanism where people can't see an obvious truth. It's also used when a person refuses to admit or face the fact they have an issue. It's been connected most prevalently with death, dying, rape and drug and alcohol addiction.

In my estimation, denial, in relationship with compulsive overeating, doesn't have so much to do with denying the issue is there, but in knowing what to do about it. Because if I admit I know what to do, then I have to do it.

Back in my super morbidly obese days, I pushed away anyone who offered me help. A friend actually told me recently that she had seen me eating candy like it was going out of style and knew I was gaining weight after losing it through surgery. She said she had wanted to say something to me.

"Why didn't you?" I asked.

"Honestly, I didn't want you to be mad at me," she said. "Would you have listened?"

I realized I wouldn't have listened. As a matter of fact, it probably would have just made me mad because I was denying I had a problem. I even refused to get on the scale. Yet, I could tell she felt guilty for not confronting me. We apologized to each other. Still I wondered, why did I deny something so evident?

Your turn. In what way has denial played a part in your weight loss process? Be specific.

Why do you think we don't want to admit to others we have a problem even though it is obvious to everyone that we do?

When have you sabotaged a process designed to help you regain your health?

Why do you think you did this?

What has to happen prior to any major effort or intervention in order for it to work?

READ AND WRITE

"For, as I have often told you before and now tell you again even with tears, many live as enemies of the cross of Christ. Their destiny is destruction, their god is their stomach, and their glory is in their shame. Their mind is set on earthly things. But our citizenship is in heaven." Philippians 3:18-20, NIV

What kinds of things cause destruction to people?

What does it mean that their god is their stomach and their glory is their shame?

How can our citizenship be in heaven if we live here on the earth in an earthly body?

ACT

Choose one person who is close to you. Share with them your desire to lose weight and ask them to help hold you accountable. Tell them specific ways they can help you. Apologize to them if you have not admitted your difficulty. Invite them to be free to speak into your life. Ask if there is anything you can help them with. Plan a time to meet, call, email, text or Facebook message them at least once a week. If you are working with a group, pair with someone from your group. Discuss your commitment level with your accountability partner. On a scale of 1 to 10, how committed are you to your accountability partner, with 1 being not committed and 10 being all in? Note this in your journal. Sign and date it.

CREATE

Draw a picture of what it means to have your stomach as your god. Share this with your group.

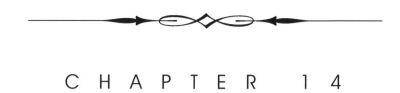

CHAPTER 14

FLIP THE SWITCH

READ CHAPTER 14, FLIP THE SWITCH

THINK ABOUT IT

"Amazing Grace" has never really been my favorite song, until Chris Tomlin came along. I love his rendition mainly for this verse: "My chains are gone. I've been set free. My God my Savior has ransomed me. And like a flood His mercy rains. Unending love. Amazing grace."

This song summarizes what happened to me in my moment of surrender. I gave up candy. It was like giving up meth or alcohol. Well, I can't say that because I've never had either of those. Sugar, though, was my addiction of choice. I never before connected the dots that I could be addicted to sugar. I thought I had to eat whatever my body craved. As freeing as it was to finally make the connection, walking it out was not all that easy. Sugar is, literally, everywhere. When you are cognizant of it, it's even more prevalent.

Have you ever thought you could be addicted to food or overeating certain foods? Why or why not?

READ AND WRITE

"All things are lawful for me, but not all things are profitable. All things are lawful for me, but I will not be mastered by anything." *1 Corinthians 6:12, NASB*

What foods control or master you? List these.

What foods do you grieve just thinking about giving them up? List these.

If giving up certain foods for the rest of your life could help you lose weight, would you do it? Why or why not?

What foods do you feel you are addicted to? Are you willing to work towards giving these foods up?

What will you give up first?

When will you start?

If you are not willing to think about giving up any food, journal about why you are hesitant.

CREATE

Write a monologue you would deliver at the service of the funeral of your favorite food. If you are working with a group, share it with them.

ACT

Go through you pantry, refrigerator and freezer and throw out all offending food items. These should be things you know are not healthy for you. If they are items family members or others think they have to have, ask them to put them somewhere you will not see them or be tempted to eat them. Make a firm decision not to purchase these items again. If others want them, they will need to purchase them and keep them where you are not tempted to eat them. Ask for their assistance in this. If they are not willing to assist you, gently let them know you have made a decision based on your health and whether or not they help, it is what you have chosen to do.

What things you will throw out, when and how?

What problems might you encounter?

How will you handle these?

How difficult will it be for you to do this?

FOLLOW-THROUGH

Journal your commitment to this process and what it was like for you to clean house, throwing out your "good friends?" Sign and date it.

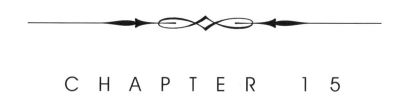

CHAPTER 15

BREAKING SWEET CHAINS

READ CHAPTER 15, BREAKING SWEET CHAINS

THINK ABOUT IT

The difficulty of family geneology is that we have to live with the hand we are dealt. Even if we were adopted or have step-parents, our biological family has a lot to do with our metabolic makeup.

I knew quite a bit about my mother's side of the family when I was required to make a genogram for a class. I knew very little about my father's side. The class was really designed for us to discover how family members interacted. Seeing it laid out on a chart back three generations helped that process.

We really weren't required to put in medical issues, substance abuse, faith or jobs but were told we could if we wanted to. For some reason, I wanted to. Being an over acheiver, I color-coded my chart. Orange was overweight and almost all had diabetes of some type. Green was alcoholism and most all were thin. The orange side was also all Christian. The green side was, for the most part, not Christian except for my father and those he had influenced. I was shocked at the sameness of color; my mother's side was all orange and dad's was all green. I saw a pattern, but I didn't know what to make of it.

Discovering that alcoholism and sugar addiction are closely related brought all the pieces of the puzzle together for me. Discovering that both sides of my family have the metabolic makeup to encourage either or both addictions was also not surprising to me.

Take a few minutes and draw a genogram. Start with yourself then your mother and father and their parents and then their grandparents. Talk to them if they are alive. If they are not alive, interview those who knew them. You can search on the internet for genogram if you are someone, like me, who likes it done right. The important thing here is to see if you can discover trends of obesity, diabetes, heart disease, alcoholism, drug abuse or other medical issues in your family lineage back at least three generations, to your grandparents. This will take you some time to do, but it will be worth it. Do it on a separate sheet of paper.

Do you see any trends? Are there a large number of those with obesity? Are their those with diabetes or other obesity related diseases? Are there those with substance abuse issues?

What does this tell you about your genetic tendencies? How does this help define what you should do?

READ AND WRITE

"Beloved, I pray that you may prosper in all things and be in health, just as your soul prospers." 3 John 2, NKJV

Why is it important that your soul prospers? What does that mean?

What does your soul need to prosper? List these.

What does your body need nutritionally to be healthy? What does it not need?

How much sleep does your body need? How much exercise does your body need?

What do you do to feed your spirit?

"But He said to me, 'My grace is sufficient for you, for My power is made perfect in weakness.' Therefore I will boast all the more gladly about my weaknesses, so that Christ's power may rest on me. That is why, for Christ's sake, I delight in weaknesses, in insults, in hardships, in persecutions, in difficulties. For when I am weak, then I am strong." 2 Corinthians 12:9-10, NIV.

How does your weakness make you strong?

How does becoming whole physically, emotionally and spiritually help break the chains of addiction?

CREATE

Find an inspiration photo from a magazine or a photo of you at the size you want to be. Write a description of what it would feel like for the current you to be this size. Attach the picture with your description to this journal.

ACT

Find an every day pair of pants and shirt, put them on and have someone take your picture with a fairly uncluttered background. Now find either an old pair of pants and shirt you would like to get into or purchase one at a garage sale, thrift store or some other place. Put the shirt and pants you wore for the picture and your new outfit in a place together. You now have your inspiration pants and shirt and can wear them for your "after" picture. If the before picture is on your phone, be sure to download it and save it on your computer or a USB drive so you will have your comparison photo.

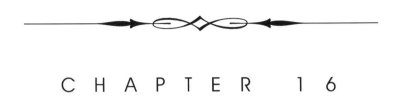

CHAPTER 16

EASY BUTTON

READ CHAPTER 16, EASY BUTTON

THINK ABOUT IT

I don't know about you, but I've gone on more diets than I can think about or even remember. The main thing I know about a diet is I always saw it as a short-term endeavor. I never saw it as something I'd do for the rest of my life.

You'd think with this type of thinking, when I'd get off track, I'd jump right back on. However, just the opposite was true. When I succumbed to temptation, I rolled over and played dead. I stopped the diet and started gaining weight again.

The thing that helped me change was to see healthy living as a lifestyle change. This doesn't mean I will do it perfect. It does mean, though, when I fail, which I surely will because none of us is perfect, I will get right back up and keep going.

Think about the times you have gotten off-track. Where did the temptation come from? Was it an internal thought process? Was it an outside person? Was it a circumstance? Was it an evil spirit? Was it a feeling? Was it a seemingly rational thought? Was it a good intention gone bad?

REFLECT

Describe a temptation to binge and how you overcome it.

When you are tempted to binge, what are some things you could do instead? List these.

READ AND WRITE

"No trial has overtaken you that is not faced by others. And God is faithful: He will not let you be tried beyond what you are able to bear, but with the trial will also provide a way out so that you may be able to endure it." 1 Corinthians 10:13, NET

Name some ways God has provided a way out of temptation for you. Did you take those ways?

"The Spirit of the One who raised Jesus from the dead is living in you. So the God who raised Christ from the dead will also give life to your bodies, which are going to die. He will do this by the power of His Spirit, who lives in you." Romans 8:11, NIRV

In what specific ways have you seen God's power at work in your life or the lives of others, especially where you knew they or you could not do it in your power alone?

ACT

Making contingency plans helps you stick with your lifestyle change. Where are some slippery places for you when you know you will be tempted to eat unhrealthy food? List these. Beside each one, write a plan to help you through those times. Note when you use the plan.

CREATE

Draw a picture using bright colored markers of how you envision the power of God. Draw yourself in the picture. What are you doing? What are you feeling? Put that feeling in the picture.

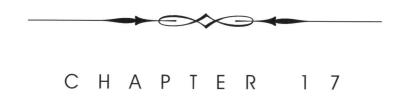

C H A P T E R   1 7

POWER FOR THE POWERLESS

READ CHAPTER 17, POWER FOR THE POWERLESS

THINK ABOUT IT

Back in the 90s Mark Lowry sang a parody he called, "I Can Eat It All." To me it was not funny. Find it on You Tube and play if you dare. The song always made me mad and then sad because I knew that person was me, but I couldn't stop myself. Apparently, many others feel that way too. Mark's song was pretty popular.

When I look at the picture of me at 430 pounds, I can feel that feeling of powerlessness over food. I can remember times I baked and ate an entire cake, two dozen cookies, the rest of the cheesy potato casserole. I felt bloated and sick. I wanted a way out. However, if you asked me if I felt powerless over food, I would have said no.

"I can stop any time I want." If you've been around any alcoholics, you've heard that said. I was in the same boat. It was extremely difficult to admit that a donut had power over me and that my life had become unmanageable, but it had.

Are you powerless over food (or any other substance)? In what ways has your life become unmanageable?

How many times have you lost and regained weight? List these times including dates, the plan you followed, how much you lost and how much you regained. Estimate if you need to. Following through with this exercise will give you a clearer picture of where you are in your journey.

Do you feel you are "insane" in the way you act regarding food or another substance? Explain your answer. Be honest.

List the ways your overeating has harmed yourself or others.

READ AND WRITE

"The Spirit of the One who raised Jesus from the dead is living in you. So the God who raised Christ from the dead will also give life to your bodies, which are going to die. He will do this by the power of His Spirit, who lives in you." Romans 8:11, NIRV

What can the power of God do? What is that one thing in your life that you secretly feel even God can't do?

ACT

Find a picture or several pictures of yourself at the weight you want to be. Copy them and paste them here. If you don't have such a picture, cut out a picture from a magazine of a person who gives you inspiration.

CREATE

Do you believe God can restore you to sanity? What would that look like? Draw a picture below representing the insane you and the sane you or write a description of each.

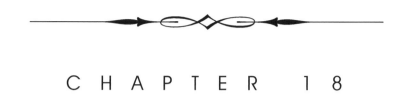

C H A P T E R   1 8

GRACE, IT'S NOT JUST A GIRL'S NAME

READ CHAPTER 18, GRACE, IT'S NOT JUST A GIRL'S NAME

THINK ABOUT IT

"I want to know and feel the smile of God on my life." At one time that was my life mission statement. It sounds really good, but it's not theological.

If I do my daily Bible reading, pray for everyone on my prayer list, visit three shut-ins, lead a small group and serve on three committees while volunteering at the hospital, I will earn God's smile, right?

Actually, if you are His child, you already have His smile. He loves you. He has plans for you that are beyond your imagination. Most likely you will only reach those if you follow His ways, but He still loves you and smiles when He sees you.

Do you agree or disagree with these statements? Why or why not?

What is the concept of cheap grace? How do we as Christians cheapen grace? What does that mean in your life?

As Christians if we sin compulsively how do you think God feels? Does He get angry with us? If not why not?

How have you been trying to earn God's smile?

READ AND WRITE

"As each of you has received a gift (a particular spiritual talent, a gracious divine endowment), employ it for one another as [befits] good trustees of God's many-sided grace [faithful stewards of the extremely diverse powers and gifts granted to Christians by unmerited favor]." 1 Peter 4:10, AMP

How can you employ grace?

ACT

List the gifts God has given you. How can you use your gifts to employ grace and further the kingdom of God?

Choose one of the ideas you listed and take one step towards doing that. If it is something simple you can accomplish completely, then do that. Journal about what the idea is, what you did and how it made you feel.

CREATE

Using photos, postcards or pictures from magazines or the internet, make a collage about the feeling or sense you have regarding God's grace. Or maybe there is just one picture that depicts grace to you. Find the picture and attach it here. Share this with your group.

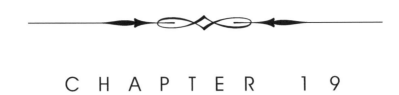

C H A P T E R   1 9

FORGIVE

READ CHAPTER 19, FORGIVE

READ AND WRITE

"Therefore, the kingdom of heaven is like a king who wanted to settle accounts with his servants. As he began the settlement, a man who owed him ten thousand bags of gold was brought to him. Since he was not able to pay, the master ordered that he and his wife and his children and all that he had be sold to repay the debt. At this the servant fell on his knees before him. 'Be patient with me,' he begged, 'and I will pay back everything.' The servant's master took pity on him, canceled the debt and let him go. But when that servant went out, he found one of his fellow servants who owed him a hundred silver coins. He grabbed him and began to choke him. 'Pay back what you owe me!' he demanded. His fellow servant fell to his knees and begged him, 'Be patient with me, and I will pay it back.' But he refused. Instead, he went off and had the man thrown into prison until he could pay the debt. When the other servants saw what had happened, they were outraged and went and told their master everything that had happened. Then the master called the servant in. 'You wicked servant,' he said, 'I canceled all that debt of yours because you begged me to. Shouldn't you have had mercy on your fellow servant just as I had on you?' In anger his master handed him over to the jailers to be tortured, until he should pay back all he owed. This is how my heavenly Father will treat each of you unless you forgive your brother or sister from your heart." Matthew 18: 23-35, NIV

Why do you think Jesus wants us to forgive? Why does it matter?

"For if you forgive other people when they sin against you, your heavenly Father will also forgive you. But if you do not forgive others their sins, your Father will not forgive your sins." Matthew 6:14-15, NIV

Does this make you more willing to forgive? Why or why not?

PROCESS

Who do you need to forgive for hurts or perceived hurts that happened in your childhood? Perceived hurts are just as real and can leave wounds that may go deep. It doesn't mean the person meant to hurt you but you FELT hurt anyway. List these.

One at time say, "I choose to forgive (insert person's name) for (insert offense)." Realize this is a process. You may need to continually affirm you have forgiven that hurt if you continue to have difficulty in that area. This is a forgiveness between you and God. It doesn't necessarily mean you need to go to the person and tell them you forgive them. But by acknowledging before God that you forgive them, you release yourself from prison and free God to begin to heal your wounds and hurts

Renounce any lie that Father God will treat you as the person you just forgave treated you. Say, "I renounce the lie that You, Father God, will (insert offense from above statement)."

Ask Father God to show you the truth He wants you to know. Ask Him to show you the truth for each lie you uncover. Say, "Father God, what is the truth?" List the truths He shows you.

Write down scriptures that support the truths of God you want to reaffirm.

If all of this seems too complicated to do by yourself, you may want to simply journal and pray about it until you feel more secure in taking this kind of prayer journey. Spend some time journaling about forgiveness, why it is important and what it means to you.

CREATE

Draw a picture of yourself and your relationship with someone you forgave. Draw how you felt before and after forgiving them. You can draw this picture even if you did not speak to them and even if they are no longer living.

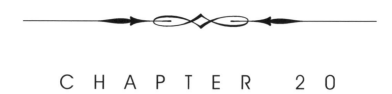

C H A P T E R   2 0

ABUNDANCE

READ CHAPTER 20, ABUNDANCE

THINK ABOUT IT

Some trips are easier to take than others. The trip through the wasteland of Kansas is always long and boring. It doesn't matter when we take it, day or night, it is the same, long, flat stretches of nothingness. On one side of that are the mountains and on the other side is my home state. So no matter what, to get to one place or the other, we have to go through Kansas.

My journey to morbid obesity was much worse than the journey back, but on both trips hrough Kansas it wasn't fun. I knew what to expect coming back, but it was still Kansas. What is God speaking to you about the journey He wants you to take?

What is your Kansas on that journey?

READ AND WRITE

"Whether you turn to the right or to the left, your ears will hear a voice behind you, saying, 'This is the way; walk in it.'" Isaiah 30:21, NIV

In what way does God show you when you have veered off the path He has for you? How do you react when He shows you? Do you immediately shut down and go the opposite way or do you use it as a learning experience? Do you turn around and go His direction?

"I have strength for all things in Christ Who empowers me [I am ready for anything and equal to anything through Him Who infuses inner strength into me; I am self-sufficient in Christ's sufficiency]." Philippians 4:13, AMP

What does this verse mean to you on your journey towards health?

"But He said to me, 'My grace is sufficient for you, for My power is made perfect in weakness.' Therefore I will boast all the more gladly about my weaknesses, so that Christ's power may rest on me. That is why, for Christ's sake, I delight in weaknesses, in insults, in hardships, in persecutions, in difficulties. For when I am weak, then I am strong." 2 Corinthians 12:9-10, NIV

How is His power made perfect in your weakness?

"Therefore, if anyone is in Christ, the new creation has come:- the old has gone, the new is here!" 2 Corinthians 5:17, NIV

In what ways are you a new creature in Christ? In what ways are you not?

CREATE

"I have come that you might have life—life in all its fullness." John 10:10b, GNB

What does abundance mean to you? Make an acrostic poem. Using the letters of the word abundance, choose a word which reminds of the attributes of that word.

A

B

U

N

D

A

N

C

E

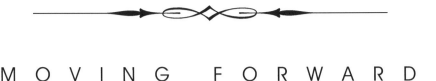

MOVING FORWARD

12 ACTION STEPS TO BEGIN YOUR JOURNEY

"For I know the plans I have for you," declares the Lord,

"plans to prosper you and not to harm you, plans to give you hope and a future,"

Jeremiah 29:11, NIV.

The Lord has plans for us. Following His way is always best. We need to make decisions about what part of His way is the most important to implement in order to get our lives back into sync, especially if we know we've gotten off track somewhere.

That was me. I had gotten off track somewhere long, long ago. I knew what was happening to me was not His plan. I took action steps to get back in line with His.

When I made the decision to do whatever it took to live, really live, even if it meant some hard work on my part, God took notice. When I actually started implementing those plans, they became easier than any diet I had ever followed. He made all of His power, that same power that raised Christ from the dead, available to me.

I still had to walk it out. I still had to say no to certain things. However, I can tell you it was the easiest hard thing I've ever done. I think part of this was the mindset shift that had happened in me as I saw one after another diet or magic fix fail.

I've boiled down the actions I took to 12 Action Steps, which have no correlation to the infamous 12 Steps.

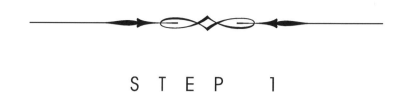

STEP 1

DECIDE TO LIVE

Most people want to live, but why do you want to live? List every reason you can think of for wanting to live. Include little things as well as big. Include things you want to do now and in the future. Include dreams you have you'd like to see come true.

Is food, or certain types of food, the only reason to live? What more to life is there than eating certain kinds of foods you love?

What type of plans does God have for you? How can you cooperate with Him to see these plans come to pass?

STEP 2

CONNECT WITH GOD

Get God's vision for your life. Invite Him to partner with you on this journey. Spend time with Him daily. Take a weekly time to stop and be quiet with Him. God wants you healthy. Know you cannot do this by yourself.

What do you do to commune with God? Circle all the ways.

Bible study

Fasting

Listening to Christian messages

Meditation

Prayer

Quiet Time

Sabbath Rest

Scripture Memorization

Talking with God throughout the day

Worship

Other _____

Extended times of solitude

Journaling

Listening to Christian music

Music and singing

Praying in the Spirit

Reading Christian books

Scripture Reading

Silence

Walking in nature

Other _____

Other _____

What is your favorite way of connecting with God? How often do you do this?

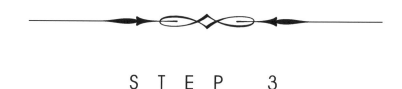

STEP 3

FIND YOUR LIFE'S PASSION

What do you do that gives your life meaning and purpose? What would you stay up late into the evening talking with friends about? What would you do if money were no object? What issues are you determined to do something about? How do you want to make a difference for others? What have you always dreamed of doing, even as a child? Why is this particular thing important to you?

What people groups are you passionate about working with?

What causes make your heart race faster?

What do you feel is your main purpose or assignment?

Why is it important for you to lose weight to fulfill this assignment?

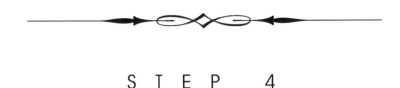

S T E P   4

STOP EATING WHAT YOU CRAVE

I craved sugar and breads. I bet you do as well. For me, the only way I could take back control was to stop eating sugar and breads. I started eating lean meats, nuts, fruits and vegetables. Sugar and carbohydrates contribute greatly to super morbid obesity, morbid obesity and obesity. We have a propensity to gain weight just thinking about something with sugar and bread. We all know those who can eat these things and not gain, but we cannot. The sooner we face this and take steps to turn away, the sooner we will start on the road to health.

What do you crave?

What foods make you grieve when you just thinking about not eating them?

Do you feel this particular food is more important than God in your life?

How will you change the way you are eating in order to lose weight?

What will you give up?

When will you start?

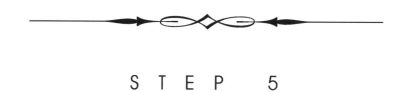

S T E P   5

DRINK MORE WATER

Stop drinking regular and diet soda. Drink at least 64 ounces of water or more a day. Many liquids, such as sodas, actually dehydrate the body. When you drink soda for instance, you are actually negating any water you drink. So the water you count bit extra liquid does not count as water and actually takes away from the water you drink.

What liquids do you drink besides water? List all of these and the amount of each you drink in a normal day. Be honest with yourself.

How can you begin to drink more water? Write down all the ways you can think of to be able to do this.

Since diet soda triggers weight gain, will you make the decision to stop drinking diet soda? How will you do this?

If you feel you need caffeine from diet soda, what will you drink instead?

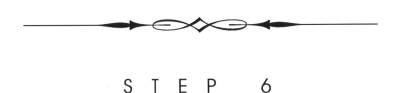

S T E P   6

DECIDE NOT TO CHEAT

Many people start on a lifestyle change, but tell themselves they will stop for the holidays or a birthday, or some other celebration. This is cheating yourself. You are making a decision to break your agreement. If you do go off your plan, go right back. Ask God to remind you of your agreement with yourself regarding your lifestyle change. Process with Him what you learn from any time you cheat.

What will be your plan to manage celebrations? Special dinners? Will you take your own food? Make special arrangements with the host? How will you go about doing this?

How will you handle eating in restaurants? What foods can be go-to foods when you eat out?

How can you learn from your mistakes? Do you need to journal, talk with a friend, pray? List what, how and when you will do this.

If you do cheat on your lifestyle eating plan, how will you make sure you get back on the plan?

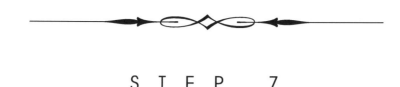

STEP 7

CHANGE YOUR MINDSET

Realize this is a lifestyle change because you have a different metabolic makeup that is more sensitive to gluten and sugar. Because of this, you cannot go back to the way you've always eaten before or you WILL gain the weight back. Changing your mindset is integral to this process. It is hard to do, but it makes the weight loss journey much easier. You have the ability to change your mindset. It is possible. You do it all the time. Remember the last time you said, "Oh that, I changed my mind." Yep, you can do it and do do it all the time!

Write down how your mind has changed regarding what you eat and how to live healthy.

What things will you do for the rest of your life?

Why are you determined to do this?

How is this time different from all of the other times you have tried to lose weight?

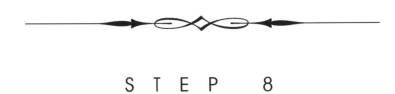

STEP 8

KEEP A FOOD JOURNAL

A food journal can be as simple as writing down items in a small notebook or with any of a number of free apps for the phone, or free programs for the computer to keep track of what you eat, your calories and exercise. I like my fitness pal, a free app for your phone and program for your computer. Whatever plan you use should be something you have with you during the day, at home, at work, at school or wherever you are.

A food journal helps you on several fronts. It helps you be accountable to yourself. It helps you understand where you might be getting off track in your eating. Seeing what you eat, the time of day, the items you eat, helps you have an overall idea of what is going on with your body. It may help you see which foods are harmful for you and which are are good for you.

Many food journal apps also have a place for you to record exercise and how many calories are burned as a result of various exercises.

What do you think will work best for you as a way to keep a food journal that includes the foods you eat, when you eat them and what their content is regarding calories, proteins and carbohydrates?

When will you start your food journal?

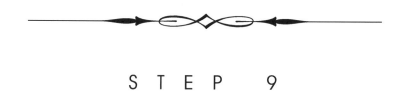

S T E P 9

EXERCISE

There are ways to exercise even if, like me, you have physical issues that limit your activity level. Various exercises include walking, aerobics, strength training, riding an exercise bike or other equipment, doing a DVD workout, doing floor or chair exercises, doing water exercise. There is really no excuse for not moving.

Why is exercise important for you?

List the exercises you are willing to do.

Where will you do these?

When will you do these?

How often will you do these?

When will you start?

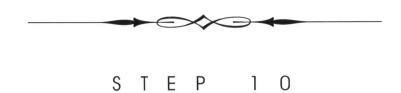

STEP 10

BE ACCOUNTABLE

Becoming a part of an accountability group and finding an accountability partner are integral steps to staying on track. Many times I would have gone backwards on my healthy eating journey had I not had a group that I knew would ask how I did that week. Not only would they ask, but if I had gotten off track they would help me process what I did wrong and how I could make a plan to make sure it didn't happen again.

Who will be your accountability partner? This can be someone further down the weight loss path than you or someone wanting to walk this same journey. If you can't find someone like that, invite someone to be your partner who believes in you and will pray for you. Invite them to hold you accountable especially if they see you slipping on your journey. What do you want from the partner and what will you give?

Write the name of your partner, when, where and how often you will meet.

How can you become a part of an accountability group, preferably led by or in participation with a life coach, counselor or psychologist who practices or agrees with cognitive behavioral therapy? List some possible groups and dates they meet. Circle the one you will go to this week.

If there is not a group, make an appointment with a counselor who can walk you through your journey. Write the name and appointment date.

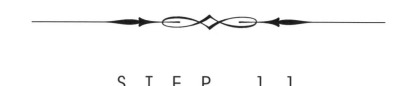

STEP 11

SEEK HOLISTIC MEDICAL ADVICE

Find a good holistic, metabolic doctor or a practitioner who believes in holistic medicine. Ask at your local health food store what local doctor or natural homeopathic practitioner helps individuals get their systems in order. Knowing what supplements to take for your stage of life and various metabolic issues can be key to your health and weight loss.

Many medical doctors simply talk about reducing calories. They do not take into consideration the myriad of difficulties women have losing weight, especially in various life stages. Simply put, a holistic doctor considers the whole person—body, emotion, mind and spirit.

For me, finding the right doctor was a major help. I do not think I would have lost the weight I did without his help. Be diligent in your search. You want someone who thinks outside the box and looks at your wellness rather than your symptoms. He or she may help you get off prescription drugs moving more towards vitamin and mineral supplements, as well as eating foods that will help maintain your body for optimal health.

This is not a practitioner who advocates the latest fad diets, but one who is serious about bringing your body systems into alignment.

Why is it important to find a holistic, metabolic doctor or practitioner?

How will you find a doctor or practitioner to help you?

When will you start? Come back and write the name and appointment date here.

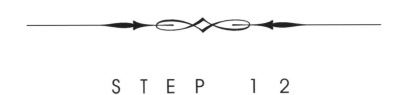

STEP 12

EAT TO LIVE DO IT AFRAID!

Those of us who have been or are currently morbidly obese know the tendency to eat to live. Sometimes it seems eating something sweet or bready is the only thing that makes getting out of bed worthwhile. However, this is certainly not true. There is so much to live for, but somehow we have gotten things turned around in our feelings which govern our priorities and, in turn, affect our behavior.

Instead of eating to live, we are living to eat whatever we want, whenever we want it. Even living to eat is a misnomer because we are really not completely living when our constant overeating causes us to develop life-threatening medical issues. Even walking into the grocery store is an effort. You long to be free of your cravings and constant desire to eat, but you are afraid to draw the line in the sand. You don't know if you can handle failing at one other weight loss plan.

If you haven't figured out by now, this is not a weight loss plan. This is the part of your life where you grab yourself by the lapels and say, "I'm not going to live this way any more. I will be healthy and I will start today with God's help. I WILL change my life. For the rest of my life I will eat healthy. No excuses. I will do this even if I have to do it afraid."

Start with any small step. Just start. Just start now, today. What will be your first step towards healthier living?

When will you take that step?

List several steps you are willing to take including when you are going to start.

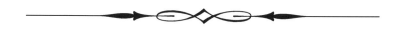

FINALE

COVENANT

Spend some time being still before God and listen to what He is saying to you, how He is gently drawing you to Himself, to come closer to walk more completely in His ways, to give up your own desires about what you want to eat. What is He saying to you? Don't guess, ask Him. Close your eyes and listen. Then, open them and write what He says here.

Even if there has been a time in your life when you have accepted Christ as your savior, have you turned everything in your life, even what you want to eat, over to God's care? Are you willing to do this or recommit to this? If so, write your commitment here.

COVENANT OUTLINE

Write out a covenant between God and yourself regarding what you have decided. Use the outline below to develop your own or adapt mine from the next page. It should be the agreement you will make between yourself and God.

Who are you and what do you wish to do? Example: I am a sugar and bread addict. I have gone to sugar and bread instead of to you, God.

Ask for His forgiveness. Example: Please forgive me for gratifying the desires of my flesh.

List the things you have hidden from others, all the places you have stored and hidden food, all the bad habits you have, all the times you know are particularly troublesome for you and give them all to Him. Example: I open every door, closet door, drawer, pantry shelf, refrigerator and freezer contents over to you. I give you my grocery shopping habits. I give you my fast food habits. I gave you every secret stash of food I have hidden in every place I know You already know about. I give You my tendency to want to eat late at night and to binge when I need an emotional fix.

Confess what you have done. Example: I confess I have gone to food instead of to You.

Surrender to Him what you are giving up. Ask Him to give you back the things you need. Example: I willingly turn this over to You. I ask that You take it all including every piece of sugar and gluten-laden items. I surrender it all to You. I ask that You give me back only those things that I should eat for my health

Ask Him to remind you when you stray. Example: I ask that You remind me each and every time I wander away from Your plan for my life.

Tell Him what you will do. Example: Right now, I covenant with you to eat lean meats, fruits, vegetables and nuts. I will to the best of my ability eat sugar-free and gluten-free.

Tell Him what will happen if you break this covenant. Example: Remind me when I break this covenant and draw me back into this covenant relationship with You, a sweet spot of grace better than any food I could eat.

Print out your covenant. Sign and date it. You may wish to display it prominently or keep it privately in a place you can refer to often.

MY COVENANT

Dear God,

I am a sugar and bread addict. I have gone to sugar and bread instead of to You. Please forgive me for gratifying the desires of my flesh.

I open every door, closet door, drawer, pantry shelf, refrigerator and freezer. I turn the contents over to you. I give you my grocery shopping habits. I give you my fast food habits. I gave you every secret stash of food I have hidden in every place I know You already know about. I give You my tendency to want to eat late at night and to binge when I need an emotional fix. I give you my desire to eat while watching television. I give you my television habits. I give you any habits where I have developed a harmful relationship with food.

I confess I have gone to food instead of to You. I willingly turn this over to You. I ask that You take it all including every piece of sugar and gluten-laden items. I surrender it all to You. I ask that You give me back only those things necessary for me to consume to become whole and healthy. I ask that You remind me each and every time I wander away from your plan for my life. I ask that when I stray You tap me on the shoulder, nudge me harder, then kick me if I don't listen. I ask that You reveal to me the underlying issue behind any time I stray, what I can learn from the incident and how I can do the right thing the next time.

Right now, I covenant with You to eat meats, fruits, vegetables and nuts. I will to the best of my ability eat sugar-free and gluten-free. Remind me when I break covenant and draw me back into this covenant relationship with You, a sweet spot of grace better than any food I could eat.

God, I turn over the secret areas of my life to Your care. I come to You realizing I need You desperately, that I am powerless to control my desire for food, especially sweets and bread, and that my life has become unmanageable. I feel insane and I believe You are the only One who can restore me to sanity by taking my hand and leading me step-by-step through this process. I make a conscious decision to turn my will and my life over to Your care. Walk with me now, God. Draw me to You through the difficult days ahead. I know it will not be easy, but it will be worth it to draw closer to You in this process, to understand more of Your amazing, unconditional love for me. I give my life totally to Your care. Amen.

—Teresa Shields Parker, May 13, 2009

SHARE

Share your decision with at least one other person or with your group. This is not an easy process. You need friends to come along side you on the road to health. Write the name of the person and the date you shared your decision with them. Share your decision with me either on my website or Facebook page. It will bless others to hear of your commitment. If you don't wish to make a public statement, please email me and tell me your decision. I want to know what God is doing in your life so I can pray with you.

THINK ABOUT IT

If you have gotten to this point it must mean you have read both *Sweet Grace* and *Sweet Grace Study Guide*. I am honored that you have taken the time to read both. I'm both happy and sad our time has come to a close. I know you have garnered some nuggets of truth to help you on your healthy living journey.

During the process of this time, you've had a lot of opportunities to think about your issues with food, sugar addiction, weight gain and loss, comfort and any myriad of other issues regarding your weight. If you have read every word in Sweet Grace, agonized over every question in the study guide, done every creative activity, completed every group activity, gone through every action step answering every question and writen, signed and dated your covenant, you must be well on your way to at least beginning your healthy living and weight loss journey.

If so, time for thinking is over. It's time to take action. God directs moving targets. Get started and then please connect with me and let me know you've started on your lifestyle change journey.

I will covenant to pray for you. I so want you to succeed, but I will not want it more than you do. That, my friend, is your job. I believe in you and I know, if I can do this, you surely can. With God on your side, there is no doubt in mind that you can and will do this!

CONNECT

If you downloaded this study guide from my website, you will receive updates about new books and products. If not, please go there and join the website in order to stay connected. Right now, to join the site, you need to download the free chapter of Sweet Grace and confirm. I know you've already read it but that's the only way to join so humor me!

I'm so glad to have shared this journey with you. Even though I don't know you personally I feel so honored that you took the time to spend with me through Sweet Grace and Sweet Grace Study Guide.

Please email me and let me know how Sweet Grace has helped you on your journey. If you share your story with me, I will not use your name unless you give me permission. I do want to share your encouraging story with others on this same healthy living journey. Your story will inspire others even if you are just starting. Please be brave and share.

One more thing and then, I'll let you peruse the photo pages, though why you'd want to I don't know. Any how, I would like you to suggest topics for my next book. I'm considering several including Change Your Mindset; Relationships and Weight Loss; Mother, Comfort and Food; Inspiration for the Weight Loss Journey; Gluten-free, Sugar-free Recipes; Weight Loss Devotional and a fiction story about a morbidly obese woman. I have ideas, I'm just wanting to know if any of these connect with you or if you'd like to hear about a different topic.

It's so hard to say Good-bye. So, connect with me so we don't have to lose touch!

CONNECT WITH TERESA

EMAIL: TERESA@WRITETHEVISION.NET

WEBSITE: TERESASHIELDSPARKER.COM

FACEBOOK: WWW.FACEBOOK.COM/TERESASHIELDSPARKERWRITER

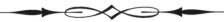

GENERATIONS

*"You saw me before I was born.
Every day of my life was
recorded in Your book.
Every moment was laid out
before a single day passed."*

Psalm, 139:16 NLT

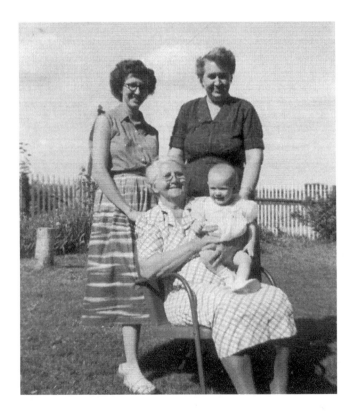

FOUR GENERATIONS—My mother, Donna Shields; my great-grandma, whom we called Mamaw, Mary White; guess who; and my grandma, Maydene Carr.

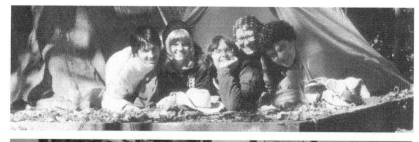

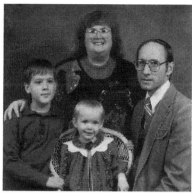

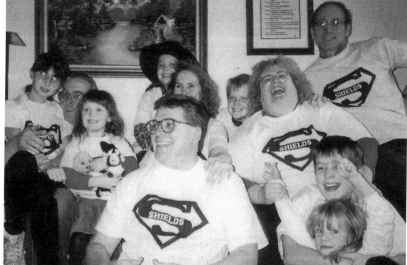

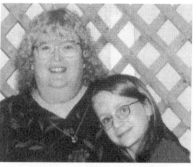

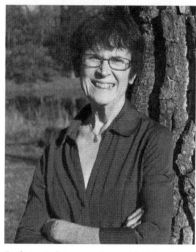

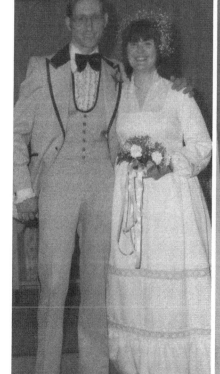

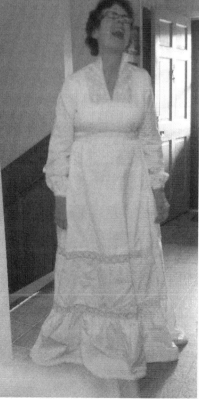

Left to right, camping with friends in Blue Ridge Mountains, 1976; Parker family, Andrew, Teresa, Jenny and Roy, 1992; Family Christmas 1995, Kristin, Dad, Nicole, Katelin, Renee, Randy, Tyler, Teresa, Jenny, Andrew, Roy; Mother's Day, 2002, Teresa and Jenny; Wedding Day, 1977 and fitting into wedding dress in 2013; Teresa, after loosing 263 pounds, 12/1/2013, determined to leave a better legacy.